Possible Errors and Weaknesses in Acupuncture Researches

I0492744

Dr. Martin Wang, MD. Ph.D.

Registered Acupuncturist
Edmonton, Canada

wenqiw57@hotmail.com

www.acupuncture123.ca

Abstract

We have found errors and mistakes in acupuncture studies in the Western countries. We now focus on analysis and discussion of improper ways of the thought, design, and performance of acupuncture studies by researchers in Western countries. We feel that, generally speaking, these researchers, due to their cultural mindset, have diverted the direction of research to understanding acupuncture as a placebo, rather than in the improvement of acupuncture performance. This has made already complex acupuncture research even more complex, causing confusion. Researchers should seek a broader view of the research area, not only expansion of his or her own research area.

Contents

Introduction 4

1. Check the reason for study failure from only one side, not both sides. ..4

2. They do not check if the acupuncture healing effect can be improved...5

3. This acupuncture is not that acupuncture 7

4. Researchers do not realize that acupuncture is highly personal skill-dependent therapy 8

5. Researchers under-estimate the difficulty of acupuncture studies.......10

6. Researchers may not be acupuncturists 11

7. Improper design of the study...11

7.1. Modified the study group to test a no-longer-natural therapy 11

7.2. Did not use simple clinic conditions to test 12

7.3. Incomplete design 12

7.4. Starting at the same time to test long-term healing effects of acupuncture...13

8. Improperly evaluating the results of the study........................13

8.1. Under-estimate the specific healing effect of acupuncture 13

8.2. Analysis on narrowed data...14

8.3. Improperly chose the population to review.........................15

8.4. Improperly using social evidence to support scientific conclusions15

Summary..16

References 17

Introduction

Acupuncture has been studied in the Western countries for more than 50 years. It is still being questioned if acupuncture has its own specific healing effect or if the observed healing effect after acupuncture treatment is only a placebo effect.[1] Previous discussion pointed out that the failure in acupuncture studies in the Western countries is mostly due to poor acupuncture healing effect derived from the acupuncture group, not so much from influence of the sham acupuncture group.[2] Here we analyze the characteristics and influence of the acupuncture researchers in Western countries on the results and conclusion of acupuncture studies.

1. Check the reason for study failure from only one side, not both sides.

The current situation in acupuncture research is that positive and negative results are published again and again even to the year 2016.[3,4,5] Most acupuncture researchers[1] paid too much attention to the sham acupuncture group, rather than checking if the acupuncture was performed in the proper way and if the healing effect has been well stimulated.

The researchers[6,7,8] suspect that the small or even no statistically significant difference between a sham and a verum acupuncture group might be due to the use of an inserted needle into the skin.[8, 9,10] The insertion might trigger or stimulate some structure to cause a reflective analgesia effect of the body.

To modify the sham group, they turned to using non-inserted sham acupuncture technique by using needles that are not inserted into the skin, or the needles that do not even touch the skin. [11,12,13,14,15] To enhance the blindness[16] of patients to the sham or verum acupuncture procedure, they chose acupuncture-naïve participants and also limited the communication of acupuncture practitioners with the patients. Due to

---

[1] The researchers in acupuncture studies may not be an acupuncturist.

the use of the sham group and for ethical compensation consideration, they may have to design a cross-over study for acupuncture. [17,18,19,20,21,22]

However, they still cannot get consistent results to tell if verum acupuncture works better than sham acupuncture.

Then the attention was also paid to ensure the equal randomization of participants by using computer-generated numbers [23] and by using sealed envelopes. [10] They used single-blind or double- or triple-blinded design.

Everything they did was designed to reduce the possible influence of the placebo effect in acupuncture studies. They avoided the use of inserted-needle sham acupuncture procedure because they worried that the inserted needle may not result in a pure placebo group (e.g. the inserted needle would cause some level of healing effect as well). To us, if we remember that our aim is to tell if typical acupuncture treatment is a placebo or not, we can still use the inserted sham acupuncture procedure. This is because of the fact that the healing effect of the inserted needle, if any, would not be too much compared with the non-inserted needle, while the study design and procedure would be much simpler compared to the current study designs with blinding and with the selection of acupuncture naïve patients. By paying more attention to using a more proper schedule for the acupuncture treatment, the difference between the verum and the sham acupuncture groups would be big enough to confirm that acupuncture has its own specific healing effect (see below). Therefore, acupuncture research could have moved forward a long time ago, and we could have avoided so many patients continuing to suffer from pain or other symptoms when they were allocated to a sham group.

2. They do not check if the acupuncture healing effect can be improved

Even if researchers have spent so much effort trying to block the influence of the placebo effect from a sham acupuncture group and a consistent result cannot be obtained, rarely is anyone questioning if the reason is due to the real acupuncture group. Surely there could be many factors affecting the efficacy of acupuncture treatment, such as how stimulating the acupuncture is in each session, the interval between treatment sessions and the total number of the treatment sessions.

In the study, it is indeed difficult to check if the acupuncture is performed in a proper way in each session, but we found that the schedule of acupuncture treatment in Western countries is different from that in China. In the former, acupuncture is performed once or twice a week and repeated in total for less than 10 to 12 times (Western style), while acupuncture in China is performed five or six times per week for more than 12 sessions (20 to 30 times; Chinese style). [2] Current data suggested that with the high treatment frequency and high total number of sessions used in China, the healing effect of acupuncture group, for most diseases tested, is high, and that in sham group, is low. [2] So the difference in the healing effect between the two groups is statistically different. Under such treatment schedule, the difference between inserted and non-inserted sham groups appeared insignificant. [24]

How come researchers in Western countries do not try the Chinese way? The researchers usually reported that they derived their acupuncture schedule from other published articles or after consulting with acupuncture experts. Just because a treatment schedule worked in another group does not mean that it is the best schedule to ensure success. It is now known that the Western style of acupuncture scheduling could yield inconsistent results – this is current situation in acupuncture research. [25] Also, the method and the schedule used by an acupuncture expert works for the expert because of his or her own personal skill but the same methods and schedule may not be suitable for a less experienced acupuncturist. An expert may use acupuncture once every three days and may only spend 10 min, but this may not be sufficient for a regular acupuncturist, no matter if the latter combines other therapies or not.

The researchers may not have checked the schedules used by acupuncturists in China in acupuncture studies. Language barrier should not be used as an excuse, since there are many acupuncture journals currently published in English too.

The researchers should also have noticed that clinical physiotherapy studies were performed mostly with more than 3 sessions per week for a total of more than 20 times, and the results were, generally speaking, positive. 2 These data should have alerted them to increasing the treatment frequency in acupuncture studies, but apparently is has not yet done so.

Why, in the acupuncture studies, is the treatment schedule in most cases only once or twice per week and less than 12 total sessions?

In communication with some researchers, they claimed that it is hard to ask Western people to participate in acupuncture every day for 20 to 30 sessions. If so, it means that the conditions necessary to start the acupuncture study have not been satisfied and it should not be launched. Is your hypothesis that acupuncture works? Or do you not care what results are gained by doing acupuncture studies this way?

3. This acupuncture is not that acupuncture

It is really hard to find out exactly how acupuncturists in Western studies performed their treatment. It has been well documented that there is a "Western medical acupuncture" [2] used in the Western countries. But what is it and is it consistent?

White A (2009) [26] introduced that "Western medical acupuncture is a therapeutic modality involving the insertion of fine needles; it is an adaptation of Chinese acupuncture using current knowledge of anatomy, physiology and pathology, and the principles of evidence based medicine. While Western medical acupuncture has evolved from Chinese acupuncture, its practitioners no longer adhere to concepts such as *Yin/Yang* and circulation of *qi*, and regard acupuncture as part of

---

[2] We feel strange that the existence of acupuncture is for medical treatment. Why do people still have to emphasize the "medical"? Is there any kind of acupuncture that is not for medical treatment?

conventional medicine rather than a complete 'alternative medical system'. It acts mainly by stimulating the nervous system, and its known modes of action include local antidromic axon reflexes, segmental and extrasegmental neuromodulation, and other central nervous system effects. Western medical acupuncture is principally used by conventional healthcare practitioners, most commonly in primary care. It is mainly used to treat musculoskeletal pain, including myofascial trigger point pain. It is also effective for postoperative pain and nausea. Practitioners of Western medical acupuncture tend to pay less attention than classical acupuncturists to choosing one point over another, though they generally choose classical points as the best places to stimulate the nervous system. The design and interpretation of clinical studies is constrained by lack of knowledge of the appropriate dosage of acupuncture, and the likelihood that any form of needling used as a usual control procedure in "placebo controlled" studies may be active. Western medical acupuncture justifies an unbiased evaluation of its role in a modern health service."

There is strong reason to suspect that many, if not all, the acupuncture performed in acupuncture studies in the Western countries belongs to such "Western medical acupuncture", rather than typical and classical Chinese acupuncture. If so, any outcomes from such Western medical acupuncture are the credit of the "Western medical acupuncture". It should not be associated with Chinese acupuncture. If it is still believed that acupuncture gives a placebo effect, then we have to make sure the results derived from Western medical acupuncture are differentiated from classical Chinese acupuncture.

It is important to acknowledge that acupuncture in Western countries might not be the same as Chinese acupuncture.

4. Researchers do not realize that acupuncture is highly personal skill-dependent therapy

Researchers do not seem to have realized that acupuncture is a highly personal skill-dependent therapy, which is similar to any other therapies that require a person to perform the treatment, such as chiropractic, massage, (or even a surgery). It does not mean that anyone who learned the theory of acupuncture knows where to insert a needle and can make the acupuncture work.

Researchers in Western studies may invite acupuncturists to perform the acupuncture, but may also invite physicians or physiotherapists to perform the acupuncture under the condition that these latter medical workers have had some hours of class education on acupuncture. We have found that more than 40% of the acupuncture was performed by physicians or physiotherapist in acupuncture studies. [25,27] We strongly suspect the personal skill of these performers who have had only 140 hours (3 weeks), [9, 27,28 ,29 ,30 ,31 ,32,33] or 10 weeks [34] of basic education in an acupuncture course before they participated the acupuncture study. In some studies, the acupuncture is even performed by students. [35] In some large-scale studies, they even did not mention the total number of acupuncturists used, nor their acupuncture training . [36,37] Sometimes, acupuncture was performed just by a non-acupuncturist, such as by a physiotherapist, [38] or by anaesthesiologists who were trained by an experienced acupuncturist.[39]

The researchers vetted the quality of the acupuncture performer by the number of years they have worked in a clinical setting only and do not have any concrete way to verify the quality of the acupuncture performer. If someone kept an acupuncture license every year but did acupuncture only one or two clients every day or every week, then how can we expect that they are as qualified in experience as typical acupuncturists who use acupuncture every day for more than 10 clients?

It is very rare that we could find an article indicating the acupuncturist's clinical success rate for a disease treatment in a study, with either acupuncture alone or acupuncture together with other therapies, such as moxibustion, cupping, bleeding therapy, and so on. If one has no experience or has a very low success rate in a natural clinic environment, then how can we show a successful rate of acupuncture treatment in a study?

The healing effect of acupuncture treatment among acupuncturists is a reality, which can be reflected in largely variable healing results by different acupuncturists in the same study.[40,41,42,43] Therefore, it can be expected that different studies with different acupuncturists could yield quite different result and that the same acupuncturists in different studies may yield similar results (success or failure).

It can be expected that, in a large-scale acupuncture study involving hundreds of acupuncture performers, with varying skill levels, the results of the study could more possibly show failure, rather than success. [31,44,45,46]

5. Researchers under-estimate the difficulty of acupuncture studies

Clinical acupuncture studies do not have the same the intensity of difficulty as clinical Western medicine (drug) studies. In the latter, the object of the study (the chemical medicine) can be standardized for its quality and quantity for testing. For example, if we want to test if Aspirin can be used to prevent coronary heart disease, the Aspirin used in US or in China would be the same in content, physical shape, color, smell or taste in each tablet. This means that the dose and quality of Aspirin give to participants is easy to control. However, this is very difficult in acupuncture. It is hard to standardize the stimulating dose of acupuncture to each patient or between treatment sessions. The tolerance of pain by each person could be different since the body condition could also be different from day to day. It is also difficult to differentiate among acupuncturists, since the personal skill of each acupuncturist is also largely different.

One of the ways to solve this problem might be to use electro-acupuncture. It can, we believe, increase the healing effect for most acupuncturists. It is could be used in a large scale study to standardize the stimulation dosage among acupuncturists and among multiple centers involved. However, it cannot completely replace the skill of an acupuncturist of master level. Also, the success of the electroacupuncture cannot completely prove that of natural and manual acupuncture.

6. Researchers may not be acupuncturists

Sometimes, we find that the acupuncture researchers in a study are not acupuncturists. The problem would be that they do not understand the difficulty of the acupuncture study (see above), so that the design of the study would not match a real acupuncture clinical environment. It would be easy to design an "artificial" or a "modified" acupuncture modality to study. Such a non-real way of acupuncture procedure could make the real acupuncturists feel frustrated and even quit the study. [47,48]

7. Improper design of the study

7.1. Modified the study group to test a no-longer-natural therapy

Acupuncture requires communication between an acupuncturist and his or her patients, to understand the feelings of the patients during treatment. The acupuncture needs to know if the Deqi sensation has been obtained and if along-meridian sensation occurs. The acupuncturist also needs to explain to the patients what acupuncture is, how it works, what may be felt during the treatment, what kind of feeling is desired and what is not desired. This is important to reduce stress and to increase confidence in the acupuncture treatment in actual clinical work environments.

However, in current acupuncture studies, communication is restricted and prevented with the aim of removing the so-called placebo effect. In the sham acupuncture group, patients not only get a sham acupuncture procedure, but also restricted communication as well. In such a study design, the acupuncture being studied is not the natural acupuncture process.

An ideal design should be to keep the acupuncture group exactly the same as in clinic environment (with communication), and in the sham group, only use sham procedure and keep other factors exactly the same as in acupuncture group (including the same way of communication).

7.2. Did not use simple clinic conditions to test

To answer if acupuncture has a placebo effect, much effort has been paid to eliminating the possible influence of a placebo effect. However, it should not be so difficult to answer this question. Placebo needs a person who is conscious so that they can believe in a hinted result. There are several clinic conditions in which the patient in unconscious, or have very mild or very weak consciousness, such as coma, shock, persistent vegetable state, being under general anesthesia, post-surgical delayed wake-up, or severe dementias. It would be hard to believe that the patients in these conditions could react to a hint and expect them to believe in hinted results. It would be straight-forward to be able to tell if acupuncture has its own specific effect in these conditions. [25] Unfortunately, there is very limited data in Western countries from studying these clinical conditions. But there is sufficient data from China to have acupuncture in such clinic conditions. To have acupuncture in such clinical conditions also allows elimination of blinding or cross-over design of the study. Surely, to have acupuncture done in such conditions need an acupuncturist of high personal skill.

7.3. Incomplete design

Someone has compared the healing effect of acupuncture by twice a week for five weeks and that done five times a week for two week. This was done by Yuan J. (2009).[49] They did not find any difference between the 2-session group and the 5-session group. However, they used moxibustion and cupping together with the acupuncture. It was a comprehensive treatment, not acupuncture alone. This can only mean that, with the combination of other therapies as in real clinical situation, the acupuncture treatment can be done twice a week. Also in this study, the healing effect in the 5-session group was better than the 2-session group in the treatment of severe cases. Moreover, the healing effect in the 2-session group saw no more improvement in the following weeks, but the treatment in the 5-session group may have continued to improve if the treatment had been continued. This means it is possible that after five weeks, the healing effect in the 5-session group might have been better than the 2-session group.

7.4. Starting at the same time to test long-term healing effects of acupuncture

There were a few studies that monitored the long-term healing effect after acupuncture treatment. They treated the patients for a fixed time period, stopped, and then monitored how the symptom level changed after a fixed time (such as 2 months, 6 months or one year). [49,50,51,52] Actually, with their acupuncture treatment, most or at least half the number of patients did not have their symptoms reduced to a minimum level. It means that the treatment only went a halfway. In a clinical situation, if the symptom were not reduced to a minimum level or to zero, the chances would be high of having a relapse of the symptoms.

We recommend starting long-term observation according to a patient's individual condition and continuing until their symptoms have been reduced to minimum (such as on a pain scale of 0-1). Meanwhile, we need to remind patients to prevent the factors that trigger or exaggerate their symptoms. For example, if the patient has lower back pain and the pain is worse when the patient lifts heavy objects (such as a nurse lifting a patient's body), we must ask them to stop lifting heavy objects. If we do not ask the patient to prevent repetition of these influencing factors, re-bound of the symptom will occur. These will contribute to the failure of the acupuncture study.

In reality, it is possible to stop acute pain with one or two applications of acupuncture and the pain can disappear for long time (can be said to be cured). However, for chronic pain, even if the pain is reduced to zero, we still need the patient to use a maintenance treatment to really fix it. Otherwise, the chance for the pain coming up again during the following observation period would be high.

8. Improperly evaluating the results of the study

8.1. Under-estimate the specific healing effect of acupuncture

Opponents of acupuncture admitted that the healing effect of the acupuncture group in a study was 10% higher than that of the sham acupuncture group. But they said that the 10% is too small and not clinically significant. The point here is that there is no evidence to suggest that the size of the placebo effect in the acupuncture group is exactly the same size of the placebo effect in the sham group. So, there is rare evidence to prove than the specific acupuncture healing effect is only 10%, rather than more than this size.[53] There are many clinical studies suggesting that, to increase the 10% healing effect in a combined therapy group, the sum of the individual therapies before combination would be much more than the total size of the combined group. Even if we take the placebo effect in the acupuncture group to be the same as in the sham group, the specific healing effect of acupuncture should be much more than the 10%. In another words, this means that to increase the 10% healing effect in the sham group, the acupuncture has to contribute much more than the 10% healing effect. Therefore, the current way of estimating acupuncture specific healing size is under-estimated.

Similarly, such under-estimation of the specific effect of an intervention in an intervention group, after subtracting the size of placebo effect from the intervention group, has been tested in drug studies. [53]

8.2. Analysis on narrowed data
Reviewers of acupuncture studies paid much attention to the surface quality of the study, such as randomization (computer-generated randomization), blind studies (single or double blind, sealed envelope), and proper size of the study (preferring large-scale studies). They collected some amount of published data, and filtered the data with these indexes to get final data for review. They believed that the data after such filtering would be so-called "high quality" data. They made summaries on these data. In many cases, they worked as a reporter, not an analyzer, of the data. Very rarely did they compare the filtered data with the whole data, or compare data published in English with data in Chinese. Since acupuncture was introduced from China, why not consider the data from China too? If the reviewer did compare the data published in the Western countries to that from China (also in English), they would not only find that the results and the conclusions are different, but also that the methods of acupuncture on both sides are also

largely different. It is not proper to refuse data just because they do not meet your index. The reviewers are usually invited by the publisher agents. The reviewer throws out so many papers for being "poorly qualified". If they are poorly qualified, then why did the journal publisher accept and allow the publication of such papers in the first place?

In the area of acupuncture studies, the reviewers never considered checking the quality of the acupuncture performer in the study and they may even not know that the acupuncture schedule in the studies in the Western countries often not the proper one.

8.3. Improperly chose the population to review

Our current question is if acupuncture has a placebo effect. We argued that the placebo effect might be less in small children and in animals. There is a review that children showed higher placebo effects than adults. However, they collected all the children from ages 0 to 12 or higher as a whole group. [54] They do not realize that children less than 1 year old might be different from those with age more than 5 or 6. Therefore, such reviewed data cannot be used to argue against the acupuncture healing effect in small children.

8.4. Improperly using social evidence to support scientific conclusions

Some researchers 1 do not believe that acupuncture has its own specific healing effect. They have even cited the personal preference of some political figures to support their scientific review results. For example, they cited that Chinese emperor Daoguan eliminated the practice of acupuncture in China, that Chairman Mao in China said that he preferred Western medicine rather than Chinese medicine, etc. We can list even more examples currently in China of people who oppose the whole of traditional Chinese medicine, including acupuncture. These people are also famous in scientific areas. They have cited side effect from Chinese medicine, but have omitted that thousands of deaths are caused by Western medicine every day. If we behave as such, we can also say that millions of people, including very famous political figures too, oppose

Christianity or Catholicism. Can we take their opinions to prove that the Christian or Catholic religions are wrong?

Every person could commit a mistake. Science needs evidence to prove hypothesis. As a researcher, we should bear scientific mind to believe evidence, not personal preference.

Summary

Scientific researchers should be open-minded. In acupuncture research, the researchers should not only understand the nature of, and specific requirement for, acupuncture treatment, but also know what is happening in similar research areas, such as in physiotherapy, chiropractice and massage, and know what has been done and how it has been done for acupuncture in China. Referring to other research areas would also help to find our own possible errors, mistakes or weaknesses in our own research areas. If researchers in Western countries did so, then acupuncture research would have moved forward much earlier to the study of the mechanism of acupuncture, rather than still be stuck in the placebo investigation and arguing if acupuncture has a placebo effect or not. Any conclusion should be carefully made if the conclusion can explain only some part of the fact or reality. Otherwise, we are technicians, not scientifically-minded researchers.

References

[1] Colquhoun D. and Steven N.
https://www.sciencebasedmedicine.org/acupuncture-doesnt-work/ Cited from Google, Aug. 1, 2015.

[2]
https://www.researchgate.net/publication/312029012_Factors_influencing_
Acupuncture_Research

[3] Fleckenstein J, Niederer D, Auerbach K, Bernhörster M, Hübscher M, Vogt L, Banzer W. No Effect of Acupuncture in the Relief of Delayed-Onset Muscle Soreness: Results of a Randomized Controlled Trial. Clin J Sport Med. 2016 Nov;26(6):471-477.

[4] Schiller J, Korallus C, Bethge M, Karst M, Schmalhofer ML, Gutenbrunner C, Fink MG. Effects of acupuncture on quality of life and pain in patients with osteoporosis-a pilot randomized controlled trial. Arch Osteoporos. 2016 Dec;11(1):34. Epub 2016 Oct 20.

[5] Feng J, Wang X, Li X, Zhao D, Xu J. Acupuncture for chronic obstructive pulmonary disease (COPD): A multicenter, randomized, sham-controlled trial. Medicine (Baltimore). 2016 Oct;95(40):e4879.

[6] Wang JJ, Wu ZH. Thinking about the conclusion of no difference between the acupuncture and sham-acupuncture in the clinically therapeutic effects on migraine abroad. Chinese Acupuncture & Moxibustion. 2009;29(4):315-319

[7] Lund I, Lundeberg T. Are minimal, superficial or sham acupuncture procedures acceptable as inert placebo controls? Acupunct Med. 2006 Mar;24(1):13-5.

[8] Lund I, Näslund J and Thomas Lundeberg T. Minimal acupuncture is not a valid placebo control in randomised controlled trials of acupuncture: a physiologist's perspective. Chinese Medicine 2009, 4:1 doi:10.1186/1749-8546-4-1

[9] Haake M, Müller HH, Schade-Brittinger C, Basler HD, Schäfer H, Maier C, Endres HG, Trampisch HJ, Molsberger A. German Acupuncture Trials (GERAC) for chronic low back pain: randomized, multicenter, blinded, parallel-group trial with 3 groups. Arch Intern Med. 2007;167(17):1892-8.

[10] Foroughipour M, Golchian AR, Kalhor M, Akhlaghi S, Farzadfard MT, Azizi H. A sham-controlled trial of acupuncture as an adjunct in migraine

prophylaxis. Acupunct Med. 2014 Feb;32(1):12-6.

[11] Park J, White A, Lee H, Ernst E: Developing of a new sham needle. Acupunct Med 1999, 17:110–112.

[12] Streitberger K, Kleinhenz J: Introducing a placebo needle into acupuncture research. Lancet 1998, 352:364–365.

[13] Takakura N, Takayama M, Kawase A, Kaptchuk TJ, Kong J, Yajima H. Design of a randomised acupuncture trial on functional neck/shoulder stiffness with two placebo controls. BMC Complement Altern Med. 2014;14:246.

[14] Zhang CS, Tan HY, Zhang GS, Zhang AL, Xue CC, Xie YM. Placebo Devices as Effective Control Methods in Acupuncture Clinical Trials: A Systematic Review. PLoS One. 2015 Nov 4;10(11):e0140825. doi: 10.1371/journal.pone.0140825. eCollection 2015.

[15] Takayama M, Yajima H, Kawase A, Homma I, Izumizaki M, Takakura N. Is Skin-Touch Sham Needle Not Placebo? A Double-Blind Crossover Study on Pain Alleviation. Evid Based Complement Alternat Med. 2015;2015:152086. doi: 10.1155/2015/152086. Epub 2015 May 7.

[16] Boutron I, Estellat C, Guittet L, Dechartres A, Sackett DL, Hróbjartsson A, Ravaud P. Methods of blinding in reports of randomized controlled trials assessing pharmacologic treatments: a systematic review. PLoS Med. 2006 Oct;3(10):e425.

[17] Pai HJ, Azevedo RS, Braga AL, Martins LC, Saraiva-Romanholo BM, Martins Mde A, Lin CA. A randomized, controlled, crossover study in patients with mild and moderate asthma undergoing treatment with traditional Chinese acupuncture. Clinics (Sao Paulo). 2015 Oct;70(10):663-9. doi: 10.6061/clinics/2015(10)01.

[18] Melchart D, Ihbe-Heffinger A, Leps B, von Schilling C, Linde K. Acupuncture and acupressure for the prevention of chemotherapy-induced nausea--a randomised cross-over pilot study. Support Care Cancer. 2006 Aug;14(8):878-82.

[19] Pfab F, Hammes M, Backer M, Huss-Marp J, et al. Preventive effect of acupuncture on histamine-induced itch: A blinded, randomized, placebo-controlled, crossover trial. J

Allergy Clin Immunol 2005;116:1386–1388.

[20] Hansen PE, Hansen JH. Acupuncture treatment of chronic tension headache--a controlled cross-over trial. Cephalalgia. 1985 Sep;5(3):137-42.

[21] Mendelson G, Kidson MA, Loh ST, Scott DF, Selwood TS, Kranz H. Acupuncture analgesia for chronic low back pain. Clin Exp Neurol. 1978;15:182-5.

[22] Petrie JP, Hazleman BL. A controlled study of acupuncture in neck pain. Br J Rheumatol. 1986 Aug;25(3):271-5.

[23] So EW, Ng EH, Wong YY, Lau EY, Yeung WS, Ho PC. A randomized double blind comparison of real and placebo acupuncture in IVF treatment. Hum Reprod. 2009 Feb;24(2):341-8. doi: 10.1093/humrep/den380. Epub 2008 Oct 21

[24] Yeung WF, Chung KF, Tso KC, Zhang SP, Zhang ZJ, Ho LM . Electroacupuncture for residual insomnia associated with major depressive disorder: a randomized controlled trial. Sleep. 2011 Jun 1;34(6):807-15. doi: 10.5665/SLEEP.1056.

[25] Wang M. https://www.researchgate.net/publication/312029059_Errors_and_mistakes _in_acupuncture_researches_in_Western_countries

[26] White A. Western medical acupuncture: a definition. Acupunct Med. 2009 Mar;27(1):33-5. doi: 10.1136/aim.2008.000372.

[27] Witt C, Brinkhaus B, Jena S, Linde K, Streng A, Wagenpfeil S, Hummelsberger J, Walther HU, Melchart D, Willich SN. Acupuncture in patients with osteoarthritis of the knee: a randomised trial. Lancet. 2005;366(9480):136-43.

[28] Linde K, Streng A, Jürgens S, Hoppe A, Brinkhaus B, Witt C, Wagenpfeil S, Pfaffenrath V, Hammes MG, Weidenhammer W, Willich SN, Melchart D. Acupuncture for patients with migraine: a randomized controlled trial. JAMA. 2005;293(17):2118-25.

[29] Brinkhaus B, Witt CM, Jena S, Linde K, Streng A, Wagenpfeil S, Irnich D, Walther HU, Melchart D, Willich SN. Acupuncture in patients with chronic low back pain: a randomized controlled trial. Arch Intern Med. 2006;166(4):450-7.

[30] Diener HC, Kronfeld K, Boewing G, Lungenhausen M, Maier C, Molsberger A, Tegenthoff M, Trampisch HJ, Zenz M, Meinert R; GERAC Migraine Study Group. Efficacy of acupuncture for the prophylaxis of migraine: a multicentre randomised controlled clinical trial. Lancet Neurol. 2006;5(4):310-6.

[31] Endres HG, Böwing G, Diener HC, Lange S, Maier C, Molsberger A,

Zenz M, Vickers AJ, Tegenthoff M. Acupuncture for tension-type headache: a multicentre, sham-controlled, patient-and observer-blinded, randomised trial. J Headache Pain. 2007;8(5):306-14.

[32] Witt CM, Jena S, Selim D, Brinkhaus B, Reinhold T, Wruck K, Liecker B, Linde K, Wegscheider K, Willich SN. Pragmatic randomized trial evaluating the clinical and economic effectiveness of acupuncture for chronic low back pain. Am J Epidemiol. 2006 Sep 1;164(5):487-96. Epub 2006 Jun 23.

[33] Witt CM, Reinhold T, Brinkhaus B, Roll S, Jena S, Willich SN. Acupuncture in patients with dysmenorrhea: a randomized study on clinical effectiveness and cost-effectiveness in usual care. Am J Obstet Gynecol. 2008 Feb;198(2):166.e1-8. doi: 10.1016/j.ajog.2007.07.041.

[34] Enblom A, Johnsson A, Hammar M, Onelöv E, Steineck G, Börjeson S. Acupuncture compared with placebo acupuncture in radiotherapy-induced nausea--a randomized controlled study.Ann Oncol. 2012 May;23(5):1353-61. doi: 10.1093/annonc/mdr402. Epub 2011 Sep 23.

[35] McKee MD, Kligler B, Fletcher J, Biryukov F, Casalaina W, Anderson B, Blank A. Outcomes of acupuncture for chronic pain in urban primary care. J Am Board Fam Med. 2013 Nov-Dec;26(6):692-700. doi: 10.3122/jabfm.2013.06.130003.

[36] Liodden I, Sandvik L, Valeberg BT, Borud E, Norheim AJ. Acupuncture versus usual care for postoperative nausea and vomiting in children after tonsillectomy/adenoidectomy: a pragmatic, multicentre, double-blinded, randomised trial. Acupunct Med. 2015 Jun;33(3):196-203. doi: 10.1136/acupmed-2014-010738. Epub 2015 Apr 13.

[37] Salter GC, Roman M, Bland MJ, MacPherson H. Acupuncture for chronic neck pain: a pilot for a randomised controlled trial. BMC Musculoskelet Disord. 2006 Dec 9;7:99.

[38] Enblom A, Lekander M, Hammar M, Johnsson A, Onelöv E, Ingvar M, Steineck G, Börjeson S. Getting the grip on nonspecific treatment effects: Emesis in patients randomized to acupuncture or sham compared to patients receiving standard care. PLoS One. 2011;6:e14766.

[39] Liodden I, Howley M, Grimsgaard AS, Fønnebø VM, Borud EK, Alraek T, Norheim AJ. Perioperative acupuncture and postoperative acupressure can prevent postoperative vomiting following paediatric tonsillectomy or adenoidectomy: a pragmatic randomised controlled trial. *Acupuncture in Medicine*. 2011;29(1):9–15

[40] Hawk C, Long CR, Rowell RM, Gudavalli MR, Jedlicka J. A randomized trial investigating a chiropractic manual placebo: a novel design using standardized forces in the delivery of active and control treatments. J Altern Complement Med. 2005 Feb;11(1):109-17.

[41] White P, Bishop FL, Prescott P, Scott C, Little P, Lewith G. Practice, practitioner, or placebo? A multifactorial, mixed-methods randomized controlled trial of acupuncture. Pain. 2012 Feb;153(2):455-62. doi: 10.1016/j.pain.2011.11.007. Epub 2011 Dec 12.

[42] Forbes A, Jackson S, Walter C, Quraishi S, Jacyna M, Pitcher M. Acupuncture for irritable bowel syndrome: a blinded placebo-controlled trial. World Journal of Gastroenterology. 2005;11(26):4040–4044. [PMC free article][PubMed]

[43] Deng G. Vickers A, Yeung S, D'Andrea GM, Xiao H, Heerdt AS, Sugarman S, Troso-Sandoval T, Seidman AD, Hudis CA, Cassileth B. Randomized, Controlled Trial of Acupuncture for the Treatment of Hot Flashes in Breast Cancer Patients. J Clin Oncol. 2007 Dec 10;25(35):5584-90.

[44] Melchart D, Streng A, Hoppe A, Brinkhaus B, Witt C, Wagenpfeil S, Pfaffenrath V, Hammes M, Hummelsberger J, Irnich D, Weidenhammer W, Willich SN, Linde K. Acupuncture in patients with tension-type headache: randomised controlled trial. BMJ. 2005;331(7513):376-82.

[45] Foster NE, Thomas E, Barlas P, Hill JC, Young J, Mason E, Hay EM. Acupuncture as an adjunct to exercise based physiotherapy for osteoarthritis of the knee: randomised controlled trial. BMJ. 2007;335(7617):436.

[46] Scharf HP, Mansmann U, Streitberger K, Witte S, Krämer J, Maier C, Trampisch HJ, Victor N. Acupuncture and knee osteoarthritis: a three-armed randomized trial. Ann Intern Med. 2006;145(1):12-20.

[47] Birch S. Reflections on the German Acupuncture studies. Journal of Chinese Med. 2007; 83: 12-17

[48] McManus CA, Kaptchuk TJ, Schnyer RN, Goldman R, Kerr CE, Nguyen LT, Stason WB. Experiences of acupuncturists in a placebo-controlled, randomized clinical trial. J Altern Complement Med. 2007 Jun;13(5):533-8.

[49] Yuan J, Purepong N, Hunter RF, Kerr DP, Park J, Bradbury I, McDonough S. Different frequencies of acupuncture treatment for chronic

low back pain: an assessor-blinded pilot randomised controlled trial. Complement Ther Med. 2009 Jun;17(3):131-40

[50] Wang Y, Xue CC, Helme R, Da Costa C, Zheng Z. Acupuncture for Frequent Migraine: A Randomized, Patient/Assessor Blinded, Controlled Trial with One-Year Follow-Up. Evid Based Complement Alternat Med. 2015;2015:920353.

[51] Avis NE, Coeytaux RR, Isom S, Prevette K, Morgan T. Acupuncture in Menopause (AIM) study: a pragmatic, randomized controlled trial. Menopause. 2016 Jun;23(6):626-37. doi: 10.1097/GME.0000000000000597.

[52] Hervik J, Mjåland O. Acupuncture for the treatment of hot flashes in breast cancer patients, a randomized, controlled trial. Breast Cancer Res Treat. 2009 Jul;116(2):311-6

[53] Lund K, Vase L, Petersen GL, Jensen TS, Finnerup NB. Randomised Controlled Trials May Underestimate Drug Effects: Balanced Placebo Trial Design. Sumitani M, ed. PLoS ONE. 2014;9(1):e84104. doi:10.1371/journal.pone.0084104.

[54] Weimer K, Gulewitsch MD, Schlarb AA, Schwille-Kiuntke J, Klosterhalfen S, Enck P. Placebo effects in children: a review. Pediatr Res. 2013 Jul;74(1):96-102. doi: 10.1038/pr.2013.66. Epub 2013 Apr 18.

Our Publications

More Than Acupuncture

Acupuncture for Emergencies

Acupuncture Styles in Current Practice

Possible Errors and Weaknesses in Acupuncture Researches

Does Nora Five-element Acupuncture Depend mostly on Psychological Effect?

Current Opinions On Shang Han Lun

Current Opinions On Classical Herbal formula systems

www.ingramcontent.com/pod-product-compliance
Lightning Source LLC
Chambersburg PA
CBHW070938220526
45468CB00005B/1812